Table of Contents

1) Introduction

Exercising in your 70's and beyond

If you're here, keep doing whatever you've been doing because it's working. Whatever physical activity you can do, do it as often as possible. If you're not already doing strength training, ask your medical providers if they can recommend any strength-training programs specifically for your age group because you can add muscle mass at any age.

If you want to enjoy an active life well into your 90s, no matter what happens NEVER STOP EXERCISING. Even if you can only do a few minutes at a time, regular exercise and physical activity can provide health benefits in every decade. If you exercise for no other reason, do it to take control of the aging process so that you can enjoy all of your favorite activities at all stages of your life.

- ## The Importance of Fitness for Seniors

Fitness is important for everyone, but it becomes even more crucial as we age. Here's why fitness is so vital for seniors:

- **Physical Health Benefits:**
  - Maintains muscle mass and strength: This helps seniors stay independent and perform everyday tasks like climbing stairs, carrying groceries, and getting out of chairs.
  - Improves balance and coordination: This reduces the risk of falls, a major cause of injury and disability in older adults.
  - Strengthens bones: This helps prevent osteoporosis and fractures.

o Boosts cardiovascular health: This reduces the risk of heart disease, stroke, and other chronic conditions.

o Manages weight: This helps prevent obesity and related health problems.

o Improves sleep quality: This can lead to better mood, energy levels, and overall health.

o Reduces joint pain and stiffness: This can improve mobility and quality of life for seniors with arthritis.

o Boosts the immune system: This helps seniors fight off infections and illnesses.

- **Mental Health Benefits:**

o Improves mood and reduces stress: Exercise releases endorphins, which have mood-boosting effects.

o Reduces symptoms of depression and anxiety: Exercise can be an effective treatment for these conditions.

o Improves cognitive function: Exercise can help maintain memory, attention, and other cognitive abilities.

o Increases self-esteem and confidence: Achieving fitness goals can boost seniors' sense of self-worth.

- **Social Benefits:**

o Provides opportunities for social interaction: Joining exercise classes or groups can help seniors connect with others and build social support.

o Reduces feelings of isolation and loneliness: Staying active and engaged can improve seniors' overall well-being.

By staying physically fit, seniors can maintain their independence, improve their quality of life, and enjoy their golden years to the fullest.

- **Overcoming Challenges and Breaking Stereotypes**

Maintaining physical fitness after 70 presents unique challenges, but also offers substantial rewards. It's crucial to acknowledge and address the common obstacles seniors face, such as managing existing health conditions, dealing with pain or fear of injury, and overcoming negative stereotypes about aging and physical capability.

Many older adults internalize societal messages that associate aging with frailty and decline, which can discourage them from engaging in physical activity. Breaking these stereotypes is essential. It's about recognizing that aging is not synonymous with inactivity and that significant improvements in strength, balance, and overall well-being are achievable at any age.

A key aspect of successful senior fitness is adapting exercises to individual needs and limitations. This might involve modifying movements, using assistive devices, or choosing low-impact activities like swimming or chair yoga. Consulting with healthcare professionals and qualified fitness instructors is invaluable for creating safe and effective exercise plans.

Finding social support through exercise groups or fitness buddies can provide motivation and accountability. Celebrating small victories and tracking progress, whether it's increased walking distance or improved balance, reinforces positive habits and boosts self-esteem.

Ultimately, overcoming challenges and breaking stereotypes surrounding senior fitness empowers older adults to take control of their health, maintain their independence, and enjoy a higher quality of life. It's about shifting the narrative around aging from one of limitation to one of possibility and continued vitality.

- **The advantages we have walking upright**

While some animals can walk upright for short periods, humans are the only mammals that are truly adapted for habitual bipedalism. This gives us several advantages:

• Greater energy efficiency: Studies have shown that humans use less energy walking on two legs than chimpanzees do when they walk on all fours. This is due to several anatomical adaptations, such as our long legs, arched feet, and unique pelvic structure.

• Long range vision: Walking upright allows us to see over tall grass and other obstacles, which would have been advantageous for spotting predators and prey in our evolutionary past.

• Free hands: Bipedalism frees our hands for carrying objects, using tools, and performing other tasks. This has been crucial for our development as a species, allowing us to create complex tools, build shelters, and care for our young more effectively.

• Improved thermoregulation: When we walk upright, we expose less of our body surface to the sun, which helps us stay cooler in hot environments. This may have been particularly important for early humans who lived in open savannas.

2. Understanding the Aging Body

• Physiological Changes in Aging

a. Musculoskeletal System:

- o Loss of muscle mass (sarcopenia): This leads to decreased strength, power, and functional capacity.

- o Decreased bone density: This increases the risk of osteoporosis and fractures.

- o Reduced joint flexibility and cartilage degeneration: This can cause pain, stiffness, and decreased range of motion.

- o Changes in posture and balance: This increases the risk of falls.

b. Cardiovascular System:

- o Decreased heart function: This can lead to reduced exercise capacity and increased risk of heart disease.

- o Stiffening of blood vessels: This can lead to high blood pressure and increased risk of stroke.

o Reduced lung capacity: This can limit oxygen intake during exercise.

c. Nervous System:

o Slower reaction time: This can affect balance and coordination.

o Impaired balance and coordination: This increases the risk of falls.

o Decreased cognitive function: This can affect motivation and adherence to exercise programs.

d. Sensory Systems:

o Vision changes: This can affect balance and coordination.

o Hearing loss: This can make it difficult to follow instructions in exercise classes.

o Decreased sense of touch: This can affect balance and coordination.

e. Metabolic System:

o Decreased metabolism: This can make it harder to maintain a healthy weight.

o Impaired glucose tolerance: This increases the risk of type 2 diabetes.

- **Common Health Concerns in Seniors**

Cardiovascular Disease: This includes heart disease, stroke, and high blood pressure. It's a leading cause of death and disability in older adults.

Arthritis: This involves joint pain and inflammation, which can limit mobility and quality of life. Osteoarthritis and rheumatoid arthritis are common types.

Osteoporosis: This condition weakens bones, making them more prone to fractures, especially in the hips, spine, and wrists.

Dementia: This is a decline in cognitive function that can affect memory, thinking, and behavior. Alzheimer's disease is the most common form of dementia.

Diabetes: This metabolic disorder affects the body's ability to regulate blood sugar. It can lead to various complications, including heart disease, kidney disease, and nerve damage.

Cancer: The risk of many types of cancer increases with age.

Respiratory Diseases: These include chronic obstructive pulmonary disease (COPD), pneumonia, and influenza.

Depression and Anxiety: Mental health concerns are common among seniors and can significantly impact their well-being.

Falls: Falls are a major cause of injury and disability in older adults, often leading to fractures and other complications.

Sensory Impairments: This includes hearing loss, vision problems (like cataracts and macular degeneration), and decreased sense of touch.

Incontinence: This involves loss of bladder or bowel control.

Oral Health Problems: This includes gum disease, tooth decay, and dry mouth.

It's important to note that these are just some of the common health concerns for seniors. Many older adults experience multiple health issues simultaneously. Regular checkups with healthcare professionals, healthy lifestyle choices, and preventive care are essential for maintaining health and well-being in later life.

- **Main obstructions to circulation**

a) Blood Circulation Obstructions:

- Atherosclerosis: The buildup of plaque (fatty substances, cholesterol, etc.) in the arteries, narrowing them and restricting blood flow. This can lead to heart attacks, strokes, and peripheral artery disease.

- Blood clots (thrombosis): Blood clots can form in veins or arteries, blocking blood flow. Deep vein thrombosis (DVT) is a clot in a deep vein, usually in the leg, while an embolism is a clot that travels to another part of the body (like the lungs, causing a pulmonary embolism).

- Vasculitis: Inflammation of blood vessels, which can narrow or block them.

- Raynaud's phenomenon: Narrowing of small blood vessels in the fingers and toes in response to cold or stress, causing temporary reduced blood flow.

b) Nerve Conduction Obstructions:

- Nerve compression: Pressure on a nerve from surrounding tissues (bone, cartilage, muscles, etc.). Examples include carpal tunnel syndrome (median nerve in the wrist), sciatica (sciatic nerve in the lower back), and pinched nerves in the neck or back.

- Nerve damage (neuropathy): Damage to nerve fibers due to various causes like diabetes, injury, infections, or autoimmune diseases. This can disrupt nerve signals.

- Tumors: Growths that can compress or invade nerves.

c) Lymphatic System Obstructions:

- Lymphedema: Blockage in the lymphatic system, often due to damage to lymph nodes or vessels (e.g., after cancer treatment). This causes fluid buildup and swelling, usually in arms or legs.

- Lymph node swelling: Enlarged lymph nodes due to infection, inflammation, or cancer. While the swelling itself isn't always a direct obstruction of flow, it indicates an issue within the lymphatic system.

d) Other Fluid Obstructions:

- Bile duct obstruction: Blockage of the tubes that carry bile from the liver to the small intestine. This can be caused by gallstones, tumors, or inflammation.

- Urinary tract obstruction: Blockage in the urinary tract (kidneys, ureters, bladder, urethra), which can be caused by kidney stones, enlarged prostate, or tumors.

- Intestinal obstruction: Blockage in the small or large intestine, which can be

caused by scar tissue, hernias, tumors, or
inflammatory bowel disease.

- Cerebrospinal fluid (CSF) obstruction:
  Blockage of the flow of CSF in the brain or
  spinal cord, which can lead to
  hydrocephalus (fluid buildup in the brain).

e) Other Types of Bodily Obstructions:

- Airway obstruction: Blockage of the
  airways in the lungs, which can be caused
  by foreign objects, swelling, or conditions
  like asthma or COPD.

- Esophageal stricture: Narrowing of the
  esophagus, which can make it difficult to
  swallow. This can be caused by scar tissue,
  tumors, or acid reflux.

It's important to note that these are just some
examples of bodily obstructions. The specific
causes, symptoms, and treatments will vary
depending on the type and location of the

obstruction. If you suspect you have any type of obstruction, it's crucial to seek medical attention for proper diagnosis and treatment.

- **Traditional Chinese Medicine (TCM)and its theories in circulation**

Traditional Chinese Medicine (TCM) places immense importance on circulation, viewing it as fundamental to overall health and well-being. The body needs unobstructed circulation to function properly. Here's a breakdown of their perspective:

Qi and Blood: The Foundation of Circulation

TCM theory centers around the concept of Qi, often translated as "vital energy" or "life force." In Western science you can also think of the Qi as nerve signal transmission. This energy flows throughout the body in specific pathways called meridians (nerve and blood pathways). Blood is considered inseparable from Qi, with Qi providing the motive force for Blood to circulate within the blood vessels. Healthy circulation, in TCM terms, means a smooth, unimpeded flow of both Qi and Blood.

The Impact of Circulation on Functioning and Activity

TCM believes that proper circulation is essential for:

- Nourishment: Blood carries essential nutrients and oxygen to all tissues and organs, while Qi ensures these substances are effectively delivered and utilized.

- Waste Removal: Efficient circulation removes metabolic waste products and toxins from the tissues, preventing their accumulation and promoting detoxification.

- Organ Function: Each organ in TCM is associated with specific functions and is reliant on adequate Qi and Blood flow to perform those functions optimally. For example, the Liver is said to "store Blood" and ensure its smooth flow, impacting menstruation, tendons, and emotional balance.

- Physical Activity: Sufficient circulation is crucial for providing energy to muscles and supporting physical exertion. When Qi and Blood flow is strong, the body can move freely and without fatigue.

- Mental and Emotional Well-being: TCM believes that the smooth flow of Qi and Blood is closely linked to emotional balance. Stagnation of Qi can lead to mood swings, irritability, and even depression.

Consequences of Poor Circulation (Blood Stasis)

In TCM, impaired circulation is often referred to as "Blood stasis." This can manifest in various ways, including:

- Pain: Especially sharp, stabbing, or fixed pain.

- Numbness and Tingling: Due to lack of nourishment to the extremities.

- Cold Limbs: Poor circulation can lead to cold hands and feet.

- Dark Complexion or Spots: Stagnant Blood can manifest as a dull or purplish complexion or the appearance of dark spots.

- Menstrual Issues: Irregular periods, painful cramps, or dark menstrual blood.

TCM Approaches to Improve Circulation

TCM utilizes various methods to promote healthy circulation:

- Acupuncture: Stimulates specific points along meridians to regulate the nervous system and Blood flow.

- Herbal Medicine: Uses herbs with properties to invigorate Blood, move energy, and dissolve stagnation.

- Tuina Massage: A therapeutic massage that manipulates muscles and meridians to improve circulation.

- Qigong and Tai Chi: Gentle exercises that promote the flow of Qi and Blood through movement and breathing.

- Dietary Therapy: Recommends foods that nourish Blood and Qi and avoid those that can contribute to stagnation.

In summary, TCM emphasizes that unobstructed circulation of Qi and Blood is fundamental for maintaining health, supporting organ function, facilitating physical activity, and promoting mental and emotional well-being. Exercise is a crucial part in gaining and maintaining unimpeded circulation throughout the body. Any pains and disfunction can be thought of as roadblocks that need to be cleared. It can also be viewed as kinks in a hose. Clearing the kinks will have an optimal flow of circulation to where it is needed.

3. The Benefits of Exercise

- Physical Benefits

Exercise provides a wealth of physical benefits that contribute to overall health and well-being. Regular physical activity strengthens the cardiovascular system, reducing the risk of heart disease, stroke, and other related conditions. Exercise improves the efficiency of the heart and lungs, enabling them to deliver oxygen and nutrients more effectively throughout the body. Furthermore, engaging in weight-bearing exercises stimulates muscle growth and increases bone density. This is particularly important for preventing osteoporosis and reducing the risk of fractures, especially in older adults. Stronger muscles also enhance functional capacity, making everyday tasks easier to perform. Exercise also plays a crucial role in improving balance and coordination. Activities that challenge balance, such as tai chi or yoga, can reduce the risk of falls, a significant concern for seniors. Finally, exercise is a cornerstone of effective weight management. It burns calories, helps maintain a healthy metabolism, and promotes a favorable body composition by increasing lean muscle mass and reducing body fat.

o Improved Cardiovascular Health

Regular exercise has a profound impact on cardiovascular health. It strengthens the heart muscle, allowing it to pump blood more efficiently with each beat. This increased efficiency lowers resting heart rate and reduces the workload on the heart. Exercise also improves blood flow and circulation throughout the body, delivering oxygen and nutrients to tissues more effectively. This improved circulation helps lower blood pressure and reduces the risk of developing hypertension. Furthermore, exercise helps improve cholesterol levels by increasing high-density lipoprotein (HDL) cholesterol, often referred to as "good" cholesterol, and lowering low-density lipoprotein (LDL) cholesterol, or "bad" cholesterol. These changes contribute to a reduced risk of atherosclerosis, the buildup of plaque in the arteries, which is a major risk factor for heart attack and stroke. Regular physical activity also improves the elasticity of blood vessels, further contributing to healthy blood pressure and reduced cardiovascular risk.

o Increased Muscle Strength and Bone Density

Exercise, particularly resistance training and weight-bearing activities, is vital for maintaining and improving muscle strength and bone density. Resistance training, which involves working against resistance using weights, resistance bands, or body weight, stimulates muscle protein synthesis, leading to muscle growth and increased strength. This increased muscle mass not only enhances physical performance but also improves metabolic health and functional capacity. Weight-bearing exercises, such as walking, jogging, and dancing, place stress on bones, which in turn stimulates bone remodeling and increases bone density. This is crucial for preventing osteoporosis, a condition characterized by weakened bones and increased risk of fractures. Stronger bones provide better support for muscles and joints, reducing the risk of injuries and improving overall mobility and stability.

o Enhanced Balance and Coordination

Regular physical activity, especially exercises that challenge balance and coordination, can significantly enhance these essential physical skills. Activities like yoga, tai chi, and Pilates focus on improving balance, posture, and body awareness, which can help prevent falls and injuries, particularly in older adults. These types of exercises strengthen core muscles, which are essential for maintaining stability and balance. Furthermore, exercises that involve complex movements and coordination, such as dancing or sports, improve neuromuscular communication, enhancing the body's ability to react quickly and efficiently to changes in position or environment. Improved balance and coordination contribute to greater confidence in movement, allowing individuals to participate in a wider range of activities and maintain their independence.

o Weight Management

Exercise plays a crucial role in weight management by creating a calorie deficit, where the body burns more calories than it consumes.

Physical activity increases energy expenditure, both during the activity itself and through an increase in metabolic rate that can persist for hours afterward. Regular exercise helps burn stored fat and maintain or build lean muscle mass. Muscle tissue is more metabolically active than fat tissue, meaning it burns more calories at rest. Therefore, increasing muscle mass through exercise can contribute to a higher resting metabolic rate, making it easier to maintain a healthy weight over time. Combining exercise with a balanced diet is the most effective approach to weight management, as it addresses both calorie intake and calorie expenditure.

- Mental Benefits
  - Reduced Risk of Cognitive Decline

Emerging research strongly suggests that regular exercise plays a significant role in reducing the risk of cognitive decline and dementia, including Alzheimer's disease. Exercise increases blood flow to the brain, delivering essential oxygen and nutrients that support neuronal function and growth. It also stimulates the release of growth factors that promote the survival and growth of new brain cells, a process known as neurogenesis. Studies have shown that exercise can improve cognitive functions such as memory, attention, and executive function, which are crucial for daily living. Regular physical activity has also been linked to a reduced risk of developing vascular dementia, a type of dementia caused by reduced blood flow to the brain.

o Improved Mood and Reduced Stress

Exercise has a powerful positive impact on mood and stress levels. During physical activity, the brain releases endorphins, which are chemicals that act as natural mood elevators and pain relievers. These endorphins contribute to feelings of euphoria, reduced stress, and improved overall well-being. Regular exercise can also help reduce symptoms of anxiety and depression. By providing a healthy outlet for stress and promoting a sense of accomplishment, exercise can improve self-esteem and confidence. Engaging in physical activity can also serve as a form of distraction from negative thoughts and worries, allowing individuals to focus on the present moment and experience a sense of mental clarity.

o Better Sleep Quality

Regular exercise can significantly improve sleep quality. Physical activity can help regulate the body's natural sleep-wake cycle, known as the circadian rhythm. Exercise can make it easier to fall asleep faster and achieve deeper, more restorative sleep. However, it's important to avoid strenuous exercise close to bedtime, as it can have a stimulating effect and make it harder to fall asleep. Regular physical activity can also reduce symptoms of insomnia and improve overall sleep efficiency, leading to more restful nights and improved daytime alertness. The mood-boosting and stress-reducing effects of exercise can also contribute to better sleep, as stress and anxiety are often major contributors to sleep disturbances.

4. Creating a Personalized Fitness Plan

Creating a personalized fitness plan is essential for maximizing results and ensuring safety.

Here's a breakdown of key steps:

- Consulting with a Healthcare Professional

Before embarking on any new exercise program, especially for individuals with pre-existing health conditions or those who have been inactive for an extended period, consulting with a healthcare professional is crucial. A physician can assess your overall health, identify any potential risks or limitations, and provide personalized recommendations based on your individual needs. This consultation may involve a physical examination, review of medical history, and discussion of any medications you are taking. A healthcare professional can also help you understand any necessary precautions or modifications to ensure your safety and prevent injuries. This step is particularly important for older adults or individuals with chronic conditions such as heart disease, diabetes, or arthritis. Other rehabilitation specialists can evaluate joint, muscle, and tendon limitations for assisted recovery and lifestyle modifications.

- Assessing Current Fitness Level

Understanding your current fitness level is a crucial starting point for creating an effective exercise plan. This involves evaluating various aspects of your physical fitness, including cardiovascular endurance, muscle strength, flexibility, and balance. Simple assessments, such as measuring your resting heart rate, performing a timed walk or run, assessing the number of push-ups or sit-ups you can do, and evaluating your range of motion in different joints, can provide valuable insights into your current fitness status. Technology can be useful while exercising to get input on your exertion levels by using a fitness watch or ring. A basic baseline for your maximum heartrate is the formula: 220-age. An example, if you are 80 years old your maximum sustained heart rate would be 140 beats per minute (bpm). Then you can adjust this rate while exercising to a sustained level of bpm depending on your health and fitness level. At the 80 yo age and having a sustained heartrate at 50% maximum would provide a guideline of 70 bpm. There are also more comprehensive fitness assessments available through fitness centers or personal trainers. By understanding your baseline fitness level, you can set appropriate goals and track your progress more effectively.

- Setting Realistic Goals

Setting realistic and achievable goals is essential for staying motivated and maintaining long-term adherence to an exercise program. Goals should be specific, measurable, attainable, relevant, and time-bound (SMART) and logged into a Fitness Journal. Instead of setting a vague goal like "get in shape," set a specific goal like "walk for 30 minutes three times a week for the next month." This makes it easier to track your progress and celebrate your achievements. It's also important to start with smaller, more manageable goals and gradually increase the intensity and duration of your workouts as your fitness level improves. Setting unrealistic goals can lead to frustration, discouragement, and an increased risk of injury.

- Choosing the Right Activities

Choosing activities that you enjoy is crucial for making exercise a sustainable part of your lifestyle. There is a wide variety of physical activities to choose from, including cardiovascular exercises like walking, running, swimming, and cycling, dancing, gardening as well as strength training, flexibility exercises, and balance training. Consider your personal preferences, interests, and any physical limitations you may have when selecting activities. It's also important to choose activities that are appropriate for your current fitness level and gradually progress as you get stronger and more conditioned. Don't be afraid to try new things and experiment with different types of exercise to find what you enjoy most. Combining different types of activities can provide a well-rounded fitness program and prevent boredom.

5. Types of Exercise for Seniors

Maintaining physical fitness after 70 is crucial for preserving independence, mobility, and overall quality of life. A well-rounded exercise program should incorporate stretching and flexibility, strength training, and endurance activities. However, it's essential to tailor these activities to individual needs and limitations, prioritizing safety, and consulting with healthcare professionals when necessary.

Overall Recommendations:

Medical Clearance: It's crucial for extremely old adults to obtain medical clearance from their physician before starting any new exercise program.

Professional Guidance: Working with a physical therapist, occupational therapist, or certified exercise specialist with experience working with seniors is highly recommended.

Start Slowly and Progress Gradually: Begin with very gentle exercises and gradually increase the intensity and duration as tolerated.

Focus on Functionality: Prioritize exercises that improve functional abilities, such as getting in and out of a chair, walking, and maintaining balance.

Monitor for Safety: Closely monitor for any signs of pain, dizziness, or fatigue, and stop the activity if necessary.

By carefully considering individual needs, adapting exercises appropriately, and seeking professional guidance, extremely old adults can safely and effectively benefit from yoga, Tai Chi, and Pilates to improve their physical function, well-being, and quality of life.

- **Flexibility and Balance**

- Stretching

General Considerations for Extremely Old Adults:

Frailty: Many extremely old adults experience frailty, characterized by decreased muscle mass, strength, and physiological reserve, making them more vulnerable to falls and other health issues.

Multiple Comorbidities: It's common for this population to have multiple health conditions, which can influence exercise choices and modifications.

Individualization: Exercise programs must be highly individualized, considering each person's unique abilities, limitations, and health status. Close supervision and guidance from qualified professionals are essential.

Stretching and Flexibility (20% of Exercise Focus)
Importance: Flexibility naturally decreases with age due to changes in connective tissues,

leading to reduced range of motion, stiffness, and increased risk of falls. Regular stretching helps counteract these changes, improving joint mobility, posture, and balance.

Recommendations: Static stretches (holding a stretch for 20-30 seconds) should be performed at least 2-3 times per week, ideally after warming up or after other forms of exercise when muscles are warm. Dynamic stretches (controlled movements through a range of motion) can be incorporated before workouts as part of a warm-up.

Duration: Each stretching session can last 10-15 minutes, focusing on major muscle groups (shoulders, back, hips, legs).

Cautions: Avoid bouncing or forcing stretches, which can lead to injury. Focus on gentle, controlled movements within a comfortable range of motion.

o Yoga

Yoga for Extremely Old Adults:

Potential Benefits:

- Improved Flexibility and Balance: Gentle yoga poses can improve joint mobility and balance, reducing the risk of falls.

- Stress Reduction and Relaxation: Yoga's emphasis on breathing and mindfulness can promote relaxation and reduce anxiety.

- Improved Sleep: Regular yoga practice may improve sleep quality.

Modifications and Cautions for extremely old people:

Chair Yoga: This adaptation of yoga uses a chair for support, making it accessible for those with limited mobility or balance issues.

Gentle Poses: Focus on simple, supported poses, avoiding inversions, deep twists, and balancing poses that could increase the risk of falls.

Qualified Instructor: A qualified yoga instructor with experience working with seniors and those with health conditions is crucial.

o Tai Chi

Potential Benefits:

Improved Balance and Coordination: Tai Chi's slow, flowing movements enhance balance, coordination, and proprioception (body awareness).

Increased Muscle Strength and Endurance: Regular Tai Chi practice can improve lower body strength and endurance.

Reduced Risk of Falls: Studies have shown that Tai Chi can effectively reduce the risk of falls in older adults.

Modifications and Cautions for extremely old people:

Simplified Forms: Shorter, simplified Tai Chi forms can be adapted for those with limited mobility or cognitive impairments.

Support: Using a chair or other support may be necessary for some individuals.

Qualified Instructor: A qualified Tai Chi instructor with experience working with seniors is essential.

o Pilates

Potential Benefits:

Core Strength and Stability: Pilates focuses on strengthening core muscles, which are crucial for posture, balance, and stability.

Improved Flexibility and Posture: Pilates exercises can improve flexibility and correct postural imbalances.

Low Impact: Pilates is generally a low-impact exercise, making it suitable for those with joint issues.

Modifications and Cautions for extremely old people:

Mat vs. Equipment: Mat Pilates may be more accessible for some individuals, while others may benefit from using specialized Pilates equipment for support.

Individualized Programs: A qualified Pilates instructor can design a program tailored to individual needs and limitations.

Qualified Instructor: Working with a qualified Pilates instructor with experience working with seniors is essential.

- **Aerobic and Endurance**

What is Aerobic Exercise and Endurance Training?

Aerobic exercise, often used interchangeably with "cardio," refers to physical activity that uses large muscle groups in a rhythmic, sustained manner. This type of exercise increases heart rate and breathing, improving the body's ability to use oxygen for energy production.

Endurance training is a type of exercise that specifically focuses on improving the body's ability to sustain physical activity for an extended period. While all aerobic exercise builds some level of endurance, endurance training emphasizes longer durations and often involves progressively increasing the duration or intensity of workouts.

How Aerobic Exercise and Endurance Training Can Be Useful for People Over 70

Aerobic exercise and endurance training offer a wide range of benefits for older adults, including:

•	Improved Cardiovascular Health: Aerobic exercise strengthens the heart muscle, improves blood circulation, and helps lower blood pressure and cholesterol levels, reducing the risk of heart disease, stroke, and other cardiovascular events

•	Enhanced Lung Function: Aerobic exercise improves lung capacity and efficiency, making it easier to breathe and engage in daily activities.

•	Increased Energy Levels: Regular aerobic exercise can combat fatigue and improve overall energy levels and helps manage weight making it easier to maintain an active lifestyle.

Endurance (Cardiovascular) Training (40% of Exercise Focus)

- Recommendations: Aim for at least 150 minutes of moderate-intensity aerobic exercise (e.g., brisk walking, swimming, cycling) or 75 minutes of vigorous-intensity aerobic exercise (e.g., jogging, hiking) per week, spread throughout the week.

- Duration: Sessions can be broken down into shorter bouts of 10-15 minutes throughout the day if needed.

- Cautions: Choose activities that are enjoyable and appropriate for individual fitness levels. Start gradually and increase the duration and intensity over time. Monitor heart rate and perceived exertion to ensure a safe and effective workout.

Specific Recommendations for People Over 70:

- Start Gradually: Begin with low-impact activities and gradually increase the duration and intensity as fitness improves.

- Choose Enjoyable Activities: Select activities that are enjoyable and motivating to promote long-term adherence.

- Consider Individual Limitations: Adapt exercises to accommodate any physical limitations or health conditions.

- Consult with a Healthcare Professional: It's important to consult with a physician before starting any new exercise program, especially for those with pre-existing health conditions.

o Walking

Description: Walking is a low-impact, accessible exercise that can be easily incorporated into daily routines. It requires minimal equipment and can be done almost anywhere.

Benefits for Seniors:

Cardiovascular Health: Regular walking strengthens the heart and improves circulation, reducing the risk of heart disease and stroke.

Bone Health: As a weight-bearing activity, walking helps maintain bone density, reducing the risk of osteoporosis and fractures.

Muscle Strength and Endurance: Walking strengthens leg muscles and improves overall endurance.

Balance and Coordination: Walking can improve balance and coordination, reducing the risk of falls.

Mental Health: Walking can improve mood, reduce stress, and enhance cognitive function.

Recommendations: Start with short walks at a comfortable pace and gradually increase the duration and intensity. Aim for at least 30 minutes of moderate-intensity walking most days of the week.

o Swimming

Description: Swimming is a full-body workout that is gentle on the joints due to the buoyancy of water.

Benefits for Seniors:

Low Impact: Swimming is ideal for seniors with arthritis or other joint problems, as it minimizes stress on the joints.

Cardiovascular Health: Swimming provides an excellent cardiovascular workout, improving heart and lung function.

Muscle Strength and Endurance: Swimming works multiple muscle groups, improving overall strength and endurance.

Flexibility: The range of motion involved in swimming can improve flexibility.

Recommendations: Start with short sessions and gradually increase the duration and intensity.

Consider taking swimming lessons or joining a water exercise class for guidance.

o Cycling

Description: Cycling, whether outdoors or on a stationary bike, is a low-impact exercise that improves cardiovascular fitness and leg strength.

Benefits for Seniors:

Cardiovascular Health: Cycling provides a good cardiovascular workout, improving heart and lung function.

Lower Body Strength: Cycling strengthens leg muscles, improving lower body strength and endurance.

Low Impact: Cycling is gentle on the joints, making it suitable for seniors with joint issues.

Recommendations: Adjust the resistance or terrain to match individual fitness levels. Start with shorter rides and gradually increase the duration and intensity. Consider using a stationary bike for added safety and stability.

o Water Aerobics

Description: Water aerobics combines aerobic exercise with the buoyancy and resistance of water.

Benefits for Seniors:

Low Impact: The buoyancy of water reduces stress on the joints, making it ideal for seniors with arthritis or other joint problems.

Cardiovascular Health: Water aerobics provides a good cardiovascular workout, improving heart and lung function.

Muscle Strength and Endurance: The resistance of water strengthens muscles without putting excessive strain on them.

Balance and Coordination: The water provides support and reduces the risk of falls, making it a safe environment to improve balance and coordination.

Recommendations: Look for classes specifically designed for seniors. Start with beginner-level classes and gradually progress to more challenging ones.

- o General Recommendations for Seniors Engaging in These Activities:

Consult with a Healthcare Professional: It's important to consult with a physician before starting any new exercise program, especially for those with pre-existing health conditions. These are general guidelines. Individual needs and abilities vary greatly.

Start Gradually: Begin with shorter sessions and gradually increase the duration and intensity as fitness improves.

Listen to Your Body: Pay attention to any signs of pain or discomfort and stop the activity if necessary.

Consistency: It is key to achieving and maintaining the benefits of exercise. Establishing a regular routine and finding activities that are enjoyable can improve adherence.

Wear Appropriate Attire and Footwear: Choose comfortable clothing and supportive footwear for walking and cycling. Wear a swimsuit and appropriate footwear for swimming and water aerobics.

Stay Hydrated: Drink plenty of water before, during, and after exercise.

Warm-up and Cool-down: <u>Always</u> include a warm-up before exercise and a cool-down afterward.

- **Strength Training (40% of Exercise Focus)**

Importance: Muscle mass and strength decline with age (sarcopenia), impacting functional independence and increasing the risk of falls and fractures. Strength training helps combat this decline, improving muscle strength, power, and bone density.

Recommendations: Strength training should be performed 2-3 times per week, with at least one day of rest between sessions to allow for muscle recovery. Focus on compound exercises that work multiple muscle groups simultaneously (e.g., squats, chair stands, push-ups against a wall, rows). Use resistance bands, light weights, or body weight as resistance.

Duration: Each strength training session can last 20-30 minutes, performing 2-3 sets of 8-15 repetitions for each exercise.

Cautions: Proper form is crucial to prevent injuries. Start with lighter weights or resistance and gradually increase as strength improves. If new to strength training, working with a qualified trainer is highly recommended. * Proper form in joint movement is the most important aspect of weight training.

Weight Training Types and Routines

o Here are some examples of strength training exercises suitable for older adults, which can be adapted using weights, resistance bands, or body weight:

• Lower Body:

Squats (or Chair Squats): Stand with feet shoulder-width apart and lower your hips as if sitting in a chair.

Lunges: Step forward with one leg and lower your body until both knees are bent at about 90 degrees.

Calf Raises: Stand with feet flat on the floor and rise up onto your toes.

Glute Bridges: Lie on your back with knees bent and feet flat on the floor. Lift your hips off the floor, squeezing your glutes at the top.

- Upper Body:

Push-ups (against a wall or on knees): Place hands shoulder-width apart on a wall or the floor and lower your chest towards the surface.

Rows (with resistance bands or light weights): Pull the resistance towards your chest, keeping your back straight.

Overhead Press (with light weights or resistance bands): Press the weight or resistance overhead.

Bicep Curls (with light weights or resistance bands): Curl the weight or resistance towards your shoulders.

Example Routine (2-3 times per week with rest days in between):

Warm-up: 5-10 minutes of light cardio (e.g., walking) and dynamic stretching.

Choose 2-3 exercises for the lower body and 2-3 exercises for the upper body.

Perform 2-3 sets of 8-12 repetitions for each exercise.

Cool-down: 5-10 minutes of static stretching.

By following these guidelines and prioritizing safety and individual needs, people over 70 can safely and effectively engage in strength training to improve their physical function, independence, and overall well-being.

Common Bodyweight Exercises (with Modifications) for oldest individuals:

o Chair Stands:

Description: Sit in a sturdy chair and stand up, then sit back down. This exercise strengthens leg muscles and improves functional strength for getting in and out of chairs.

Modifications: If standing up is difficult, use armrests for support or start with a higher chair. As strength improves, gradually reduce reliance on armrests or lower the chair.

o Wall Push-ups:

Description: Stand facing a wall, place hands shoulder-width apart on the wall, and lean in until your elbows are bent. Push back to the starting position. This exercise strengthens chest, shoulder, and arm muscles.

Modifications: Adjust the distance from the wall to modify the difficulty. Standing closer to the wall makes the exercise easier.

o Calf Raises (with Support):

Description: Stand holding onto a sturdy chair or countertop for support and rise up onto your toes, then lower back down. This exercise strengthens calf muscles and improves balance.

Modifications: Perform the exercise while seated if standing is difficult.

o Hip Extensions (Standing or Lying):

Description:

Standing: Hold onto a sturdy chair or countertop and extend one leg straight back behind you, squeezing your glutes.

Lying: Lie on your stomach and lift one leg straight up off the floor, squeezing your glutes.

Modifications: Limit the range of motion if needed.

o Side Leg Raises (Standing or Lying):

Description:

Standing: Hold onto a sturdy chair or countertop and lift one leg out to the side.

Lying: Lie on your side and lift the top leg up towards the ceiling.

Modifications: Limit the range of motion if needed.

o Knee-to-Chest Stretch:

Description: Lie on your back and bring one knee towards your chest, holding it with your hands. This exercise improves hip and lower back flexibility.

Modifications: Perform the stretch while seated if lying down is difficult.

- Adjusting exercise routines as you age over 70

I had already suggested the guidelines for the percentages of time in doing each routine with:

Flexibility training at 20%

Endurance training at 40%

Strength training at 40%

These guidelines are generally for people in their 70's and in good health. But, these guidelines should be adjusted for those people who are in their 8th, 9th, decades and beyond in living. As people are getting older in these decades, more emphasis should be given to circulation and joint mobility. You should still do all three aspects of training if you can but more of your training will be devoted to flexibility and stretching training. Of course, these guidelines would be adjusted on an individual basis.

o People in their 80's:

Flexibility training at 40% - 50%

Endurance training at 30% - 25%

Strength training at 30% - 25%

o People in their 90's and beyond:

Flexibility training at 50% - 60%

Endurance training at 25% - 20%

Strength training at 25% - 20%

6. Lifestyle Factors for Optimal Health

• Nutrition

Nutrition: A Cornerstone of Healthy Aging and improve exercise outcomes

Nutrition plays a vital role in maintaining health and well-being throughout life, but it becomes especially critical for senior citizens.

As we age, physiological changes occur that can affect nutrient absorption, metabolism, and overall nutritional needs. Adequate nutrition is essential for maintaining physical function, cognitive health, immune function, and overall quality of life in older adults.

- o Physiological Changes Affecting Nutritional Needs in Seniors:

Decreased Metabolism: The metabolic rate tends to slow down with age, meaning seniors require fewer calories to maintain their weight. However, their need for essential nutrients remains the same or even increases.

Reduced Digestive Function: Changes in the digestive system can affect nutrient absorption, making it important to consume nutrient-dense foods.

Decreased Sense of Taste and Smell: These sensory changes can reduce appetite and food intake, potentially leading to nutrient deficiencies.

Changes in Body Composition: Muscle mass tends to decrease with age (sarcopenia), while body fat may increase. Adequate protein intake is crucial to preserve muscle mass.

- o Chronic Health Conditions: Many seniors have chronic health conditions that can affect their nutritional needs and dietary restrictions.

Medications: Some medications can interact with nutrients or affect appetite, requiring dietary adjustments.

- Essential Nutrients for Seniors

Protein: Adequate protein intake is essential for maintaining muscle mass, immune function, and wound healing. Good sources include lean meats, poultry, fish, eggs, beans, lentils, and dairy products.

<u>Calcium, Magnesium, and Vitamin D</u>: These nutrients are crucial for bone health and preventing osteoporosis. Fortified foods, and sunlight exposure are good sources of calcium and vitamin D.

While dairy products can be a good source of calcium and vitamin D, there are some reasons why older people might need to limit or avoid them:

Lactose Intolerance: Lactose is a sugar found in milk and other dairy products. Lactase is an enzyme in the small intestine that helps digest lactose. As people age, they produce less lactase, making it harder to digest lactose. This can lead to bloating, gas, diarrhea, and other digestive issues after consuming dairy.

Weakened Immune System: Some dairy products, like soft cheeses made from unpasteurized milk, can harbor harmful bacteria. Seniors with weakened immune systems are more susceptible to infections from these bacteria.

Medication Interactions: Dairy products can interfere with the absorption of certain medications.

Other Health Conditions: Some seniors may have health conditions that require them to limit or avoid dairy, such as:

Heart Disease: Dairy products can be high in saturated fat and cholesterol, which can raise the risk of heart disease.

Prostate Cancer: High dairy consumption has been linked to an increased risk of prostate cancer in some studies.

Hormone related cancers: Dairy products contain natural growth hormones which can increase the risk of certain cancers.

- Here are some excellent non-dairy sources:
  - Calcium:

<u>Leafy Greens:</u>

Kale: A cup of cooked kale provides about 10% of the daily recommended value of calcium.

Collard Greens: One cup of cooked collard greens offers over 25% of the daily recommended value.

<u>Bok Choy</u>: This leafy green is also a good source of calcium, along with other vitamins and minerals.

<u>Fortified Plant-Based Milk:</u>

Almond Milk, Soy Milk, Rice Milk: Many plant-based milk alternatives are fortified with calcium and vitamin D, making them comparable to cow's milk in terms of these nutrients. Check the nutrition label to ensure they are fortified.

Tofu: Tofu that is processed with calcium sulfate is a good source of calcium.

Canned Fish with Bones:

Sardines and Salmon: These fish are rich in calcium because they contain edible bones. They also provide omega-3 fatty acids, which are beneficial for heart health.

Other Sources:

Almonds: A handful of almonds provides a decent amount of calcium.

Figs: Dried figs are a good source of calcium and fiber.

Oranges: Oranges contain some calcium, and fortified orange juice is a good source.

o Magnesium:

Leafy Greens:

Spinach: A half-cup of cooked spinach provides a significant amount of magnesium.

Swiss Chard: Another excellent source of magnesium, as well as other nutrients.

Nuts and Seeds:

Almonds, Cashews, Pumpkin Seeds: These are all good sources of magnesium.

Legumes:

Black Beans, Kidney Beans: Beans and lentils are good sources of magnesium, fiber, and protein.

Whole Grains:

Brown Rice, Quinoa: Whole grains provide magnesium along with other important nutrients.

Avocados: Avocados are a good source of magnesium and healthy fats.

Dark Chocolate: Dark chocolate (with a high cocoa content) contains magnesium and antioxidants.

Vitamin B12: Vitamin B12 absorption can decrease with age. Fortified foods and supplements may be necessary to ensure adequate intake.

Fiber: Fiber promotes digestive health, helps regulate blood sugar levels, and can lower cholesterol. Good sources include fruits, vegetables, whole grains, and legumes.

Healthy Fats: Healthy fats, such as those found in avocados, nuts, seeds, and olive oil, are important for brain health and overall well-being.

- Hydration:

Staying hydrated is crucial for seniors, as dehydration can lead to various health problems. Seniors should drink plenty of water throughout the day, even if they don't feel thirsty.

- Meal Planning and Preparation

Plan Weekly Menus: Creating a weekly menu can help ensure a balanced intake of nutrients and make grocery shopping easier.

Consider Nutrient Density: Focus on nutrient-dense foods that provide a lot of nutrition in smaller portions. This is important because seniors often have smaller appetites.

Incorporate Favorite Foods: Include familiar and enjoyable foods to encourage appetite and meal satisfaction.

Plan for Leftovers: Cooking larger portions and using leftovers for future meals can save time and effort.

Use Visual Aids: Use pictures or written lists to help with meal planning, especially for those with memory problems.

Involve Seniors in the Process: Include seniors in meal planning and grocery shopping as much as possible to promote independence and engagement.

o Meal Preparation Strategies:

Simplify Recipes: Choose simple recipes with fewer ingredients and easy-to-follow instructions.

Use Convenience Foods Wisely: opt for pre-cut vegetables, canned beans, and other convenience foods to reduce preparation time and effort, but be mindful of sodium and added sugars.

Batch Cooking: Cook larger batches of food and freeze individual portions for easy reheating on busy days or when energy levels are low.

Use Kitchen Gadgets: Utilize kitchen gadgets such as slow cookers, food processors, and microwaves to simplify meal preparation.

Modify Food Textures: If chewing or swallowing is difficult, modify food textures by chopping, mashing, or pureeing foods.

Create a Comfortable Eating Environment: Ensure a comfortable and pleasant eating environment to encourage appetite and meal enjoyment.

o Addressing Specific Needs:

For Seniors with Limited Mobility:

Consider grocery delivery services or assistance from family or friends.

Use assistive devices such as reachers and jar openers.

Arrange the kitchen for easy access to frequently used items.

o For Seniors with Cognitive Impairments:

Use visual cues and reminders for meal preparation.

Prepare meals in advance and store them in easy-to-access containers.

Consider meal delivery services or assistance from caregivers.

o For Seniors with Limited Budgets:

Plan meals around affordable staples such as beans, rice, and pasta.

Utilize coupons and discounts at grocery stores.

Consider participating in community meal programs or food banks.

o Socialization and Mealtime:

Encourage Social Dining: Eating with others can improve appetite and make mealtimes more enjoyable.

Participate in Community Meal Programs: Many senior centers and community organizations offer congregate meal programs that provide nutritious meals and social interaction.

By implementing these meal planning and preparation strategies, seniors can maintain a healthy diet, improve their overall well-being, and promote independence.

- **Sleep**

Sleep is a fundamental physiological need that plays a vital role in physical and mental health at all ages, but it's particularly important for older adults. While sleep patterns may change with age, the need for quality sleep remains. Adequate sleep is essential for:

<u>Cognitive Function</u>: Sleep plays a crucial role in memory consolidation, learning, and cognitive performance. Poor sleep can contribute to memory problems, difficulty concentrating, and increased risk of cognitive decline.

<u>Physical Health</u>: Sleep is essential for physical repair and restoration. It supports immune function, cardiovascular health, and metabolic

regulation. Poor sleep can increase the risk of chronic diseases such as heart disease, diabetes, and obesity.

<u>Emotional Well-being</u>: Sleep deprivation can lead to mood swings, irritability, anxiety, and depression. Adequate sleep promotes emotional stability and overall well-being.

<u>Fall Prevention</u>: Poor sleep can impair balance and coordination, increasing the risk of falls, a significant concern for older adults.

   o Common Sleep Changes in Older Adults:

<u>Changes in Sleep Architecture</u>: Older adults often experience changes in sleep architecture, including a decrease in deep sleep and an increase in lighter sleep stages. This can lead to more frequent awakenings during the night and a feeling of less restful sleep.

<u>Changes in Circadian Rhythm</u>: The body's internal clock (circadian rhythm) can shift with

age, leading to earlier bedtimes and earlier wake-up times.

<u>Increased Prevalence of Sleep Disorders</u>: Older adults are more likely to experience sleep disorders such as insomnia, sleep apnea, and restless legs syndrome.

o Tips for Better Sleep for People Over 70:

<u>Establish a Regular Sleep Schedule</u>: Go to bed and wake up at the same time each day, even on weekends. This helps regulate the body's natural sleep-wake cycle.

<u>Create a Relaxing Bedtime Routine</u>: Develop a relaxing bedtime routine that includes activities such as taking a warm bath, reading a book, or listening to calming music.

<u>Optimize the Sleep Environment</u>: Ensure the bedroom is dark, quiet, and cool. Use comfortable bedding and pillows.

<u>Limit Daytime Naps</u>: If you nap during the day, keep them short (20-30 minutes) and avoid napping late in the afternoon.

<u>Avoid Caffeine and Alcohol Before Bed</u>: These substances can interfere with sleep.

<u>Regular Physical Activity</u>: Regular exercise can improve sleep quality but avoid strenuous exercise close to bedtime.

<u>Manage Medications</u>: Review medications with a physician to identify any that may be interfering with sleep.

<u>Address Underlying Health Conditions</u>: Treat any underlying health conditions that may be contributing to sleep problems, such as pain, sleep apnea, or restless legs syndrome.

<u>Consider Cognitive Behavioral Therapy for Insomnia</u> (CBT-I): CBT-I is a structured program that helps individuals identify and change

negative thoughts and behaviors that contribute to insomnia.

<u>Consult a Healthcare Professional</u>: If sleep problems persist, it's important to consult with a physician or sleep specialist to rule out any underlying medical conditions or sleep disorders.

By prioritizing sleep hygiene and addressing any underlying sleep problems, people over 70 can significantly improve their sleep quality and reap the many benefits of restful sleep for their physical and mental health.

- **Stress Management**

While exercise itself is a powerful stress reliever, unmanaged stress can significantly hinder an exercise and fitness program for older adults in several ways:

Decreased Motivation and Adherence: When stressed, individuals may experience low energy, lack of motivation, and difficulty concentrating, making it challenging to stick to an exercise routine. Stress can also lead to procrastination and avoidance of physical activity.

Increased Risk of Injury: Stress can lead to muscle tension, decreased coordination, and impaired judgment, increasing the risk of falls and other injuries during exercise.

Impaired Recovery: Chronic stress can interfere with the body's ability to recover from exercise, leading to muscle soreness, fatigue, and an increased risk of overtraining.

Negative Impact on Sleep: Stress can disrupt sleep patterns, which can further exacerbate fatigue and hinder exercise performance. Poor sleep also impairs muscle recovery and overall well-being.

<u>Exacerbation of Existing Health Conditions</u>: Stress can worsen existing health conditions such as heart disease, arthritis, and diabetes, which can limit exercise capacity and increase the risk of complications.

- Integrating Stress Management into Exercise Programs:

It's crucial to integrate stress management techniques into exercise programs for older adults to maximize benefits and minimize risks. Here are some strategies:

  o Relaxation Techniques

Before or After Exercise: Incorporate relaxation techniques such as deep breathing exercises or gentle stretching before or after workouts to reduce muscle tension and promote relaxation.

<u>Deep Breathing Exercises</u>: Practicing deep, slow breaths can help calm the nervous system and reduce stress.

<u>Progressive Muscle Relaxation</u>: This technique involves tensing and releasing different muscle groups in the body to promote relaxation.

<u>Guided Imagery</u>: This involves visualizing calming scenes or situations to reduce stress and promote relaxation.

<u>Warm Baths or Showers</u>: Soaking in warm water can help relax muscles and reduce tension.

o Mindfulness and Meditation

<u>Mindful Exercise</u>: Focus on the present moment during exercise, paying attention to your breath, body sensations, and the movements you are performing. This can enhance the stress-reducing benefits of exercise.

<u>Mindfulness Meditation</u>: This practice involves focusing on the present moment without judgment, helping to reduce stress and improve attention.

<u>Yoga and Tai Chi</u>: These gentle forms of exercise combine physical movement with mindfulness and breathing techniques to promote relaxation and stress reduction.

o Social Connection

<u>Social Support</u>: Exercise with a friend, family member, or in a group to provide social support and motivation.

<u>Choose Enjoyable Activities</u>: Choose activities you find enjoyable and motivating, as this can help reduce stress and improve adherence.

<u>Stress Management Education</u>: Provide education on stress management techniques and encourage seniors to incorporate these techniques into their daily lives.

<u>Adapt Exercise Intensity</u>: During periods of high stress, it may be necessary to reduce the intensity or duration of workouts to avoid overtraining and injury.

<u>Prioritize Sleep Hygiene</u>: Emphasize the importance of good sleep hygiene and encourage seniors to establish a regular sleep schedule and create a relaxing bedtime routine.

By recognizing the impact of stress on exercise and integrating stress management techniques into fitness programs, older adults can maximize the benefits of physical activity and improve their overall health and well-being.

7. Overcoming Obstacles and Staying Motivated

Maintaining an active lifestyle becomes increasingly important with age, yet individuals over 70 often face unique challenges that can hinder their engagement in regular exercise. Addressing these obstacles and fostering motivation are crucial for long-term adherence and realizing the numerous physical and mental health benefits of physical activity.

- Dealing with Pain and Injury:

Pain and the fear of injury are significant deterrents to exercise for many older adults. It's essential to distinguish between normal muscle soreness after exercise and pain that indicates a potential injury.

Listen to Your Body: Encourage seniors to pay close attention to their bodies and stop any activity that causes sharp or persistent pain.

Consult Healthcare Professionals: If pain persists or an injury occurs, prompt consultation with a physician or physical therapist is crucial. They can diagnose the issue, recommend appropriate treatment, and provide guidance on modified exercises or rehabilitation.

Modify Exercises: Adapt exercises to accommodate physical limitations or existing conditions. This may involve reducing the range of motion, using assistive devices, or choosing low-impact alternatives.

Proper Warm-up and Cool-down: Implementing a thorough warm-up before exercise and a cool-down afterward can help prevent injuries and reduce muscle soreness.

- Overcoming Fear and Intimidation:

Many older adults may feel apprehensive about starting or resuming an exercise program, particularly if they have been inactive for an extended period or have concerns about their physical capabilities.

Start Gradually: Encourage a gradual approach to exercise, beginning with low-intensity activities and slowly increasing the duration and intensity over time.

Choose Appropriate Activities: Select activities that are enjoyable, accessible, and appropriate for individual fitness levels and preferences.

Seek Professional Guidance: Working with a qualified fitness professional experienced in working with older adults can provide personalized guidance, demonstrate proper form, and offer encouragement and support.

Focus on the Benefits: Emphasize the numerous benefits of exercise for older adults, including improved physical function, reduced risk of falls, enhanced mood, and increased independence.

- Finding a Fitness Buddy:

Social support can play a vital role in maintaining motivation and adherence to an exercise program.

Exercise with a Partner: Encourage seniors to find a friend, family member, or neighbor to exercise with. Having a workout partner can provide motivation, accountability, and social interaction.

Join Group Exercise Classes: Participating in group exercise classes or senior fitness programs can provide a sense of community and support.

Utilize Community Resources: Many senior centers, community centers, and fitness facilities offer programs specifically designed for older adults.

- Tracking Progress and Celebrating Successes:

Tracking progress and celebrating achievements can significantly enhance motivation and reinforce positive exercise habits.

Set Realistic Goals: Encourage seniors to set specific, measurable, achievable, relevant, and time-bound (SMART) goals.

Keep a Fitness Journal: Tracking workouts, progress, and any challenges encountered can provide a sense of accomplishment and help identify areas for improvement.

Use Fitness Trackers or Apps: Wearable fitness trackers or smartphone apps can help monitor activity levels, track progress, and provide motivation.

Celebrate Milestones: Acknowledge and celebrate achievements, no matter how small they may seem. This can reinforce positive behavior and encourage continued participation.

By addressing these obstacles and implementing strategies to foster motivation, individuals over 70 can successfully engage in regular exercise and reap the numerous physical and mental health benefits of an active lifestyle.

8. Conclusion

- The Power of Aging Actively

In closing, we've explored the profound impact of active aging for those over 70, a time of life often mistakenly associated with decline rather than opportunity. This book has aimed to dispel those myths, offering practical strategies and insights to empower you to embrace this chapter with vitality and purpose. We've delved into the multifaceted benefits of physical activity, from strengthening muscles and bones to boosting cognitive function and enhancing emotional well-being. We've examined the importance of nourishing your body with proper nutrition, prioritizing restorative sleep, and effectively managing stress—all crucial components of a holistic approach to healthy aging.

It's vital to remember that aging actively is not about striving for an unrealistic ideal of youth. It's about optimizing your current health and well-being, maximizing your independence, and finding joy and fulfillment in each day. It's about adapting activities to your individual needs and abilities, celebrating small victories, and recognizing that progress, not perfection, is the ultimate goal.

The power of aging actively resides within each of you. It's about making conscious choices to prioritize your health, engage in meaningful activities, and maintain connections with others. It's about challenging limiting beliefs and embracing the potential for continued growth and vitality. This is not just about adding years to your life, but adding life to your years.

We encourage you to use the information and strategies presented in this book as a guide, but most importantly, to listen to your own body and intuition. Consult with healthcare professionals when needed, seek support from family and friends, and find activities that bring you joy and purpose.

The journey of aging is a unique and personal one. By embracing the principles of active aging, you can navigate this journey with confidence, resilience, and a deep appreciation for the richness and possibilities that this stage of life offers. The power to age well is in your hands—embrace it.

With love!

Brian P Kramer

SOURCES

Is Walking Upright an Adaptation to Beat the Heat? - Lam Museum of Anthropology - lammuseum.wfu.edu

Warm up and cool down activities | NHS inform - www.nhsinform.scot

Resistance training – preventing injury - Better Health Channelwww.betterhealth.vic.gov.au

Older Adults and Balance Problems | National Institute on Aging - www.nia.nih.gov

How Functional Training Improves Everyday Movement And Mobility -functionaltraininginstitute.com

The Key Role of Physical Activity in Longevity - Welbrook Memory Care

Role of nutrition in performance enhancement and postexercise recovery - PubMed   Central - pmc.ncbi.nlm.nih.gov

Talking With Your Older Patients | National Institute on Aging

Electrocardiogram (ECG) - NHS - www.nhs.uk

Blood Pressure Assessment in Adults in Clinical Practice and Clinic-Based Research: JACC Scientific Expert Panel - PMC - PubMed Central - pmc.ncbi.nlm.nih.gov - medlineplus.gov

LDL and HDL Cholesterol and Triglycerides – CDC - www.cdc.gov

Benefits of Physical Activity – CDC - www.cdc.gov

How can strength training build healthier bodies as we age? | National Institute on Aging - www.nia.nih.gov

Why Should Senior Citizens Perform Balance Exercises? - Freedom Care - freedomcare.com

Osteoporosis and exercise - Better Health Channel - www.betterhealth.vic.gov.au

Physical Activity and Your Heart - Benefits | NHLBI, NIH - www.nhlbi.nih.gov

Review Article: Sarcopenia: Causes, Consequences, and Preventions - Oxford Academic - academic.oup.com

Low Bone Density > Fact Sheets > Yale Medicine - www.yalemedicine.orgAging changes in the bones - muscles - joints: MedlinePlus Medical Encyclopedia -

medlineplus.gov

Fall Prevention: Balance and Strength Exercises for Older Adults | Johns Hopkins Medicine - www.hopkinsmedicine.org

Cardiovascular Considerations in the Older Patient – Physiopedia - www.physio-pedia.com

www.americansportandfitness.com

24ssuissenews.net

Benefits of Physical Activity – CDC - www.cdc.gov

Physical Inactivity and Cardiovascular Disease - New York State Department of Health - health.ny.gov

Exercise and Lung Health | American Lung Association - www.lung.org

Train Smarter, Not Harder: Personalized Fitness Sessions for You - Prime Health - www.primehealthandperformance.com

Talk With Your Doctor Before Starting A New Exercise - TRUE Fitness - shop.truefitness.com

The Annual Checkup: Why Regular Health Assessments Matter - Advanced Medical P.A. - www.wellingtonadvancedmed.com

Exercise safety - Better Health Channel - www.betterhealth.vic.gov.au

What is a fitness assessment and how can you benefit from it? - wellness.nifs.org

Aging, Nutritional Status and Health – PMC - pmc.ncbi.nlm.nih.gov

Nutrition needs when you're over 65 - Better Health Channel - www.betterhealth.vic.gov.au

Hydration Status in Older Adults: Current Knowledge and Future Challenges – PMC - pmc.ncbi.nlm.nih.gov

Dehydration, Cognitive Functioning, & ADLs - GuideStar Eldercare - guidestareldercare.com

Healthy Meal Planning: Tips for Older Adults | National Institute on Aging - www.nia.nih.gov

Overcoming Barriers to Elderly Exercise - Aegis Living - www.aegisliving.com

How Physical Therapy Can Diagnose and Treat Nerve Pain - amberhillpt.com

Injured? Hold the Ice and Start Moving | For Patients - Dartmouth Health - www.dartmouth-health.org

Boosting Physical Activity among Older Adults: Strategies for Senior Centers - www.ncoa.org

Personal Training for Seniors: 5 Benefits - Holbrook Life - holbrooklife.com

What Do We Know About Healthy Aging? - www.nia.nih.gov

Embracing a Healthy Lifestyle for a Better You - Prime Plus Medical -www.primeplusmed.com

Four Types of Exercise and Physical Activity - National Institute on Aging - www.nia.nih.gov

Fueling Your Body: The Role of Nutrition in Overall Health - Saint Mary's Health Network - saintmarysreno.com

Making Sleep a Priority for Mental Well-Being - American Psychiatric Association - www.psychiatry.org

Frailty in Older Adults: Evidence for a Phenotype - Oxford Academic - academic.oup.com

Exercise Can Help Decrease Fall Risk for Elderly People - School of Medicine - medicine.tufts.edu

Yoga Instructor Explains Breathing Techniques | Piedmont Healthcare - www.piedmont.org

Yoga for Sleep | Johns Hopkins Medicine - www.hopkinsmedicine.org

Chair Yoga: Gentle Exercises for Seniors with Limited Mobility - Banner Health - www.bannerhealth.com

Centers for Disease Control and Prevention (CDC): "Physical Activity Basics"
https://www.cdc.gov/physicalactivity/basics/index.htm

World Health Organization (WHO): "WHO guidelines on physical activity and sedentary behaviour"
https://www.who.int/publications/i/item/9789240015128

Is Dairy Good or Bad for Aging Adults? Are Dairy Products Healthy or Unhealthy for the Elderly? - Home Care Oshkosh

seniorstridehomecare.com

Lactose Intolerance | Johns Hopkins Medicine - www.hopkinsmedicine.org

Lactose malabsorption and intolerance in older adults – PMC - pmc.ncbi.nlm.nih.gov

The Importance of Sleep for Seniors - SRG Senior Living - www.srgseniorliving.com

Aging and Sleep: How Does Growing Old Affect Sleep? | Sleep Foundation - www.sleepfoundation.org

Sleep's Crucial Role in Preserving Memory - Yale School of Medicine - medicine.yale.edu

Impact of Sleep on the Risk of Cognitive Decline and Dementia - PMC - PubMed Central - pmc.n

What is the relationship between physical activity and chronic pain in older adults? A systematic review and meta-analysis protocol - PMC - PubMed Central - pmc.ncbi.nlm.nih.gov

Brian Kramer, MS, is a practitioner of Oriental Medicine, Biologist, and Fitness Trainer.

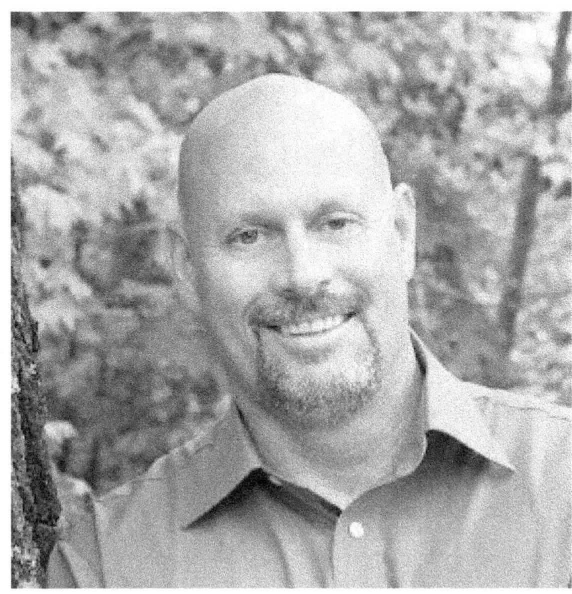

For decades, Brian Kramer has been helping people improve their health and wellness through combinations of natural remedies and therapies. He is an advocate of the idea that "Exercise is Medicine" and designing personalized fitness routines for his patients and clients. He has been an athlete and fitness enthusiast most of his life. In his teen years, he was a marathon cyclist and continued playing basketball for over 20 years. After a short tour in the U.S. Coast Guard, he discovered a love for Natural Body Building and Nutrition which drove his passion for gaining more of an understanding of how the body works. This gave him a drive for learning more about Human Anatomy and Physiology which led to him obtaining a bachelor's degree in biology from the University of New Mexico while beginning a Fitness Training and Sports Nutrition business.

As Brian gained more knowledge and experience about health and wellness, he wanted to find a deeper understanding of how to help people be healthy and not merely treating illness. He discovered Oriental Medicine as an important means in achieving balance in health and wellness through the approaches of acupuncture, herbal medicines, nutrition, and physical rehabilitation strategies. He graduated from Southwest Acupuncture College in Albuquerque New Mexico with a Master's in Oriental Medicine. He then moved to Raleigh North Carolina and has had a thriving clinical practice and fitness training business.

Brian loves being in nature and finding time to engage in hiking adventures, and camping all over the country while pulling his small pop-up camper.

NOTES

NOTES